KETO DIET

& INTERMITTENT FASTING SUCCESS

Discover the Simple Steps to Cleanse the Body of Toxins, Balance Hormones, and Promote Weight Loss

JERRY ADATSI

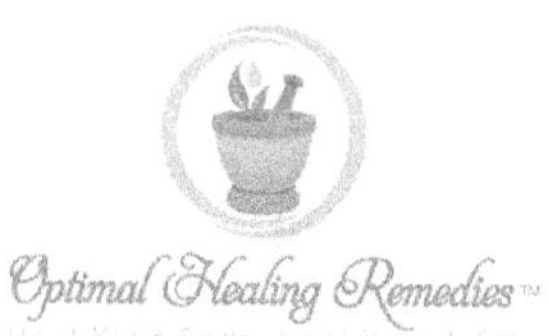

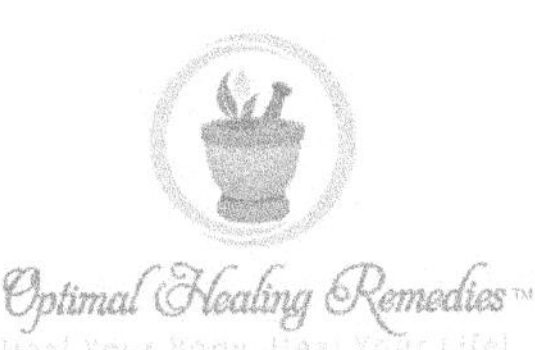

Under no circumstances will any blame or legal responsibility be held against the author, or publisher, for any damages, reparation, or monetary loss due to the information within this book, either directly or indirectly.

<u>Disclaimer Notice:</u>

Please note the information within this document is for educational and entertainment purposes only. All effort has been executed to present accurate, up to date, reliable, and complete information. No warranties of any kind are declared or implied. Readers acknowledge that the author is not engaged in the rendering of medical, legal, financial or professional advice. The content within this book has been derived from various sources. Please consult a licensed medical professional before attempting any techniques outlined in this book.

By reading this document, the reader agrees that under no circumstances is the author responsible for any losses, direct or indirect, that are incurred because of the use of the information within this document, including, but not limited to, errors, omissions, or inaccuracies.

Table of Contents

CHAPTER 1

INTRODUCTION

UNDERSTANDING THE KETOGENIC DIET AND INTERMITTENT FASTING

Intermittent fasting and ketogenic diets have cemented a place amongst the health trends in recent times. The immense benefits of these two dietary concepts to individuals' overall well-being necessitate writing a book on both topics. As you will discover in this book, intermittent fasting and keto diets provide remarkable health benefits for you—on both physical and mental planes. Even those who are knowledgeable in this area will find the book interesting, as it contains verifiable facts and a straightforward approach to implementing these concepts in your life.

THE BASICS OF INTERMITTENT FASTING

The term intermittent fasting is used to describe a variety of eating schedules centered on alternating between fasting and feeding. It is not about regulating what you eat; rather, the essence of intermittent fasting is to control when you eat. Intermittent fasting follows a daily window where eating is allowed at predefined times. A time is set for eating, while the remaining time is a non-eating period. For instance, individuals may eat only at particular times of the day, like 11:00 am and 5:00 pm. During the fasting period, it may be permissible to drink a predetermined amount of water to keep your body hydrated. However, snacks are not permitted since the essence is to regulate the intake of calorie-containing food.

Intermittent fasting has been a human practice to heal the body for centuries. It has historically been used as a therapeutic process for a wide range of ailments and health conditions, such as obesity, diabetes, and epilepsy. Some people unintentionally practice this process by intentionally skip meals, often doing this for days at a stretch. Such individuals, while purposefully skipping food intake, may not know he or she is practicing intermittent fasting. When the body experiences food and calorie scarcity, it becomes sensitive to insulin. This is very important because insulin levels ensure that calories from food are used up by the body or stored for future use.

Individuals engaged in weight-altering and muscle-building procedures have also embraced intermittent fasting as an effective regimen to achieve their desired results. It should be understood that intermittent fasting is a healthy procedure, with benefits including better brain functioning and cancer prevention.

In the modern era, however, the prevalence of factory-manufactured foods has changed many people's eating habits because the majority of our diets are now sure recipes for varying degrees of health problems. While intermittent fasting is an age-old tradition, the science behind it has exposed people to the benefits. Some have observed that when individuals fast, they allow their bodies to go through a natural cleansing process while their systems embark on the regeneration and repair process to function optimally. Intermittent fasting is a behavioral intervention that helps to synchronize the body's rhythms for improved hormonal regulation to optimize the overall health of the human body.

THE BASICS OF THE KETOGENIC DIET

The human body is built so that when glucose is available, it uses it as fuel for energy. With excess glucose remaining after fueling the body's needs, the excess is converted to fat that is subsequently stored up as reserves, which could be used if a prolonged period of glucose shortage occurs in the body.

However, maybe the body also depletes the stored glucose, leaving the system with no glucose reserve to serve the energy needs of the body. This is called ketosis and is described as a metabolic state characterized by a depletion of reserve glucose in the body. It is ideal for the reduction of body fat and for balancing the glucose level inside the blood.

Human physiology has been programmed to be reluctant to burn fats in the body. With this in mind, sometimes missing out on a meal will not result in the human body entering ketosis and burning fat. When the body is in a ketonic state, the consumption of too many carbohydrates will switch off ketosis by putting the body back into a fat-storage mode. Anyone who wants to attain ketosis should know the nutrient requirements necessary to enable this state and ensure that the body meets this required level. This varies from person to person since everyone is not performing the same daily energy-sapping activities.

The ketogenic diet is based on what you eat, with little or no emphasis placed on when you eat. For starters, a generally acceptable macronutrient percentage to achieve an effective state of ketosis will follow the proportion given below:

- at most, 10% of daily calories from carbohydrates
- at most, 30% of daily calories from protein-based food
- 60% or more of daily calories from fat-based food

There is a misconception that fat is bad in any diet; hence, a daily diet containing over 60% of dietary fat is considered by some to be hazardous. However, dietary fat differs from body fat, and carbohydrates are more complicit in increasing body fat than fat from your diet.

When considering the ketogenic diet as a long-term solution, some experts recommend that a cyclical approach yields the greatest benefit. With a cyclical ketogenic diet, high-carb intake is allowed two days out of the week. For example, the keto practitioner replaces feeding periods covering 5 days with two days of increased carb intake. It is believed that this process allows your metabolism to reset.

THE BENEFITS OF COMBINING INTERMITTENT FASTING WITH THE KETO DIET

People have often asked if it is possible to combine these two processes into one. The answer to this is yes, it is possible. While the two standalone processes share a common end result—ketosis—combining the two creates a powerful and effective dietary regimen for fat reduction. To get a better perspective of why combining both is more effective than just one method, you only need to understand how each works. Intermittent fasting is focused on <u>when</u> you eat while keto diet deals with <u>what</u> you eat.

By combining the two, the results will be amplified. One important benefit is that it helps the body reduce the negative side effects of ketosis. For instance, when the body is shifting from glucose to ketone production, some people do experience keto flu. Mind you, it is not flu in the real sense, nor is it infectious—it is merely a body condition that takes the form of flu, with symptoms including headaches, fatigue, dizziness, sugar cravings, and lack of motivation.

By changing your eating pattern towards keto-based food and keeping to a particular eating time window, you can simply eat without feeling as if you have eaten too much.

By following a regimen that combines both, you will discover that eating keto-friendly foods will make you feel satiated; hence, when you begin intermittent fasting, you don't put your mind towards food because you will not feel hunger pangs.

Also, a combination of the keto diet and intermittent fasting gives the practitioner mental clarity—your body feels satiated, your energy levels are high, and you lose weight. All of these combined give a feeling of greatness and achievement. What a way to kick off a full keto diet and to acclimate you to the concept of food abstinence! If you are unsure which one to embrace, combining the two will work well as they complement each other without putting particular strains on the individual. It may take serious discipline to practice both. However, you can be sure that it is worthwhile because the result outweighs the sacrifice you put into it.

~ 8 ~

CHAPTER 2

BODY CLEANSING WITH KETO AND INTERMITTENT FASTING

CLEANSING THE BODY WITH INTERMITTENT FASTING

Detoxification is the process of eliminating the toxins within the body, especially in strategic areas such as the colon, liver, lungs, skin, and lymph nodes. Cleansing the body can be done in one of two ways—through the ingestion of antibiotics or through a natural process called autophagy. Autophagy is regarded as the most effective way to rejuvenate cells in the body. Imagine the process like a garbage disposal that occurs naturally at the cellular level. During this process, the dysfunctional parts of the human cells are obliterated, so they have no harmful effect on the body as a whole. The autophagy process can be triggered by limiting food intake. It also helps the body to destroy pathogens while building a stronger immune system.

One major benefit of intermittent fasting is that it precipitates this detoxification process of autophagy since food is no longer entering the body. In the absence of food, the body kicks off the process of self-cleansing to neutralize or eliminate toxins. Autophagy ensures that the body cleanses and recycles cells it perceives as not functioning properly. Through this, the immune system is boosted, which ultimately prevents diseases that result in quick aging. Calorie restriction caused by intermittent fasting counteracts the accumulation of damaged and old cells in the body, thus enhancing the metabolic efficiency of healthy cells in the body, which slows down the aging process.

Intermittent fasting helps increase the connections within the hippocampus in the brain. This area is associated with mood, memory, and motivation and also has neuron-protecting attributes. By engaging in intermittent fasting, recovering from brain injuries and the promotion of mental acuity and focus is possible. The human digestive system is put to rest, leading to immense benefits that include more energy and stamina, a clearer skin tone, and clarity of mind.

A study by Saad and Elnemr in 2009 on the effects of intermittent fasting during Ramadan and Lent indicated increased metal detoxification of the body. Researchers collected samples from male volunteers, and results showed a reduction of zinc in the blood after persistently fasting for over 25 days. Also, there was a significant decrease in selenium levels in the blood, while toxic agents such as lead, cadmium, and manganese also decreased within the same period. Studies have also shown that intermittent fasting is a great way to slow the progression of cancer cells in the body since detoxification takes place during the period of continuous fasting. Intermittent fasting also regulates inflammation levels in the body by clearing the antigenic cells and triggering the immune response necessary for reducing inflammation.

CLEANSING THE BODY WITH THE KETO DIET

Another effective and natural process to cleanse the body is through biotransformation, which eliminates toxins from the body. Biotransformation transforms toxic material into benign molecules that can be expunged from the system through sweat, urine, or feces. This process requires ingesting certain vitamins and minerals and other nutrients to handle the increase of toxic agents in the body.

To allow biotransformation to take place effectively, incorporate foods with the capacity to support the process, including cruciferous vegetables like broccoli and dandelions. One way to cleanse the body with the keto diet is to limit the consumption of calorie-dense foods with little nutritional value, like highly processed foods.

By substituting them for detox diets that contain more plants and herbs, the body can eliminate toxins that have accumulated in the body for some time. A good keto diet will not only provide the body with nutrients that improve immune system performance but also ensure that toxic agents are broken down into forms that can be easily removed from the system.

A keto diet allows the body to produce lysosomes, a garbage disposal-like structure that helps to break down old and faulty proteins in the body. Ketogenic diets are rich in healthy fats and proteins and mimic the effects of fasting by producing ketone bodies. The ketone bodies are very efficient at cleansing the body by switching on a mechanism called chaperone-mediated autophagy (CMA), a process that recycles cellular waste. This provides an effect similar to someone fasting due to the metabolic changes that occur.

Recent studies have revealed that brain tumor cells are, to a large degree, dependent on glucose for growth. With a keto diet, the tumor cells are starved of the necessary glucose; hence, they die off. It encourages the body to burn more fats that may hold on to toxins. The activation of Nrt2, an antioxidant path responsible for turning up the detoxification process of cellular in the body, also ensures the improvement of gut barrier integrity of the body.

PRACTICAL STEPS FOR DETOXIFYING WITH KETO AND INTERMITTENT FASTING

Detoxifying with the keto diet and intermittent fasting include a combination of food abstinence and careful meal selection that will aid the objective. Without keto diets and intermittent fasting, the liver and kidneys would automatically detoxify the body. This covers you to some extent. But when the toxin level within the body increases due to fat being burned by the body, these two organs may become overworked since they are not equipped with the power to convert and expunge such large deposits of toxins. Detoxification through a keto diet and intermittent fasting has interrelated steps that ensure the effective removal of toxins from the body.

The first step in detoxifying the body through a keto diet is to ensure that the foods you're eating are sourced from the cleanest and highest-quality grades. Non-organic foods and meat and dairy products may contain pesticides and other synthetic hormone residues that affect the body's hormonal balance and detoxification process. Exposure to antibiotics often triggers insulin resistance in the body. This may lead to severe alteration of the gut microbiome (Klancic and Reimer, 2020). Therefore, limiting exposure to harmful chemicals by choosing organic animal products is important.

Although keto diets are very rich in fat and protein, a larger proportion of dietary fat should not come from bad fats like hydrogenated vegetable oils, margarine, trans fats, oils made from soy, corn, cottonseed, canola, or excessive animal protein. The keto diet should be comprised of foods with non-saturated fats, like seeds, olives, avocados, and nuts. Fat from red meat may also inhibit toxins from being released from the body, which makes detoxification difficult. It is better to focus on fat from fish and seafood, like wild caught Alaskan Salmon and Sardines. It is also advisable to stay away from artificial sweeteners that may be keto-friendly but hinder the body from embarking on a natural detoxification process.

It is equally important to support the gut with fiber and probiotics. Detoxification needs a robust gut microbiome. The benefit of this is that the gut bacteria break down various compounds, including mycotoxins and hormones. Detoxification can be impaired when environmental toxins disrupt the healthy balance of bacteria inside the gut. That is why it is important for your keto diet to be rich in fiber to boost resilience to toxins. Another benefit of dietary fiber is that it enhances the functionality of the intestinal proteins, which is a strategic part of detoxification. Probiotic supplements also assist in detoxifying environmental chemicals within the body.

Frequent Hydration

For proper detoxification to take place, you must drink plenty of water. People on keto diets often overlook adequate hydration as an essential part of detoxification. However, drinking lots of high-quality water whenever you feel thirsty will help the kidney and intestinal tracts to easily embark on detoxification. The optimal water intake will depend on factors such as age, body size, climate, and activity level.

Toxic Binding

The moment toxins have been separated from the fat tissues, they need to be "mopped up" quickly, so they don't get redistributed back into the tissues again. While on a keto diet, it is also good to make use of binding agents such as bentonite clay or activated charcoal. These binding agents are very efficient at absorbing toxins released from the body by the fat tissues, then excreting them out. However, remember each identified binding agent's has particular toxins that they work with; bentonite clay absorbs metal toxins and mycotoxins while activated charcoal works best for bacterial toxins.

Improve Liver Functionality

There are a variety of ways to naturally improve liver functionality during keto dieting. For instance, milk thistle is a traditional botanical medicine used for centuries to treat liver disorders like hepatitis. Recent research has also demonstrated that silymarin, a major component of milk thistle, protects the liver against dangerous chemicals and supports ketosis. Also, vegetables rich in sulfur, like cruciferous vegetables and alliums such as onions and garlic, support detoxification.

To speed up the detoxification process, some supplements naturally support keto diets. For example, natural supplements such as Vitamin D3, Magnesium, Medium-chain triglycerides (MCT) oils, electrolytes, and dark-green vegetable powders can be very beneficial. By consuming such supplements, you can avoid experiencing negative side effects when your body enters the ketogenic state. For individuals with underlying health conditions, seek expert medical advice before starting a keto diet and intermittent fasting for detoxification.

Chapter 3

Balancing Hormones With Keto and Intermittent Fasting

Balancing Hormones With the Keto Diet

Hormones play an important role in the body; they have a great effect on mental health and the emotional and physical states of the body. Hormonal secretion also impacts body weight, mood, and mental output, amongst other things.

Keto diets help balance the body's hormonal levels while also treating hormone disorders. Recent studies have discovered that the keto diet improves insulin response and results in positive changes in the hormone levels now prevalent in modern society that contribute to various health issues. Keto diets help balance hormones by improving the performance of insulin in the body. Recently, there has been a rise in issues related to insulin resistance, but the majority of those concerned are often unaware of the problem. They find out that their major problem originated from insulin resistance only when they begin to experience chronic health issues.

Keto diets also affect cortisol, a hormone constantly released by the adrenal glands in the body. The adrenal glands release hormones into the bloodstream and also respond to other hormonal secretions and chemicals in the body. The adrenal glands may become exhausted when faced with an excess of glucose (resulting from consuming too many carbohydrates). This causes the blood sugar to fluctuate rapidly, leading to a stressed response from the adrenal glands. By frequently consuming ketogenic foods, the adrenal glands feel less stress, resulting in improved regulation of cortisol metabolism. One way to balance the hormone level in the body is to reduce carbohydrate intake, which ultimately results in lowering insulin levels so that the hormonal level of the body is balanced.

One common problem caused by hormone imbalance is polycystic ovary syndrome (PCOS), a hormonal disorder that causes enlarged ovaries with noticeable cysts at the edge. This disorder often leads to infertility in women. While the prevalence of this disorder is low, keto diets have come far in correcting such hormonal imbalances. Although there is no known cure for PCOS, a good keto diet accompanied by keto-friendly supplements gets PCOS under control. Researchers from Duke University also discovered that women suffering from PCOS who followed the advice of a prolonged keto diet balanced their insulin levels while also experiencing improvements in infertility, menstruation, and other gender-specific problems.

 To support this, Cabeca and Gilberg-Lenz (2019) advised that keto dieting is the perfect diet for women going through major hormonal changes or increased hormone fluctuations. They further stated that ketogenic nutrition assists women in fixing their hormones, so they can keep themselves healthy as they age. Balancing the hormone levels of the body is possible with a keto diet that includes low-level carbohydrate foods, such as citrus drinks, fermented and probiotic foods, cruciferous vegetables, and sesame seeds.

BALANCING HORMONES WITH INTERMITTENT FASTING

Intermittent fasting has been confirmed to be an effective means of balancing hormones in the body if it is done correctly. However, this regimen does not work for men and women in the same way because the female biological makeup responds to situations like fasting differently than that of males.

One way that intermittent fasting balances the hormone levels in the body is by reducing insulin resistance. This situation leads to the cells in the body not effectively recognizing insulin (which acts as a glucose-storing hormone). In women, however, this may lead to fertility complications such as PCOS. If it is done properly, intermittent fasting increases insulin sensitivity, helping the body fight against type 2 diabetes and PCOS. It also helps in supporting the body's fat-burning mechanisms that improve weight loss.

Intermittent fasting also leads to increased growth hormones. These hormones are necessary for burning fat and repairing the muscle mass of the body. The growth hormones increase the utilization and availability of fats to energize the body. When you eat as soon as you wake up and continue to snack throughout the day, there is little opportunity for growth hormones to activate and engage in muscle repairs. However, with intermittent fasting, you allow the growth hormones to repair muscles. In 2016, Jason Fung noted that over a five-day fasting period (full water only fast or intermittent fasting), the growth hormones in the body would double.

Intermittent fasting engages another hormone-balancing activity, the reduction of cortisol and subsequent increase in melatonin secretion. While cortisol is a stress hormone, melatonin is secreted by the body to induce sleep.

Melatonin is secreted to help you fall asleep and allow the body to rest and feel invigorated when you wake up. By engaging in a nutrient timing schedule paired with intermittent fasting, the result is a well-balanced combination of cortisol and melatonin release to provide the optimal energy and mental awareness needed to start the day.

Intermittent fasting also aids in the increased secretion of adiponectin, which is necessary for the burning of bad fats. This, with reduced insulin resistance, lowers the blood sugar levels in the body. Intermittent fasting has also been confirmed to increase new neuron formation in the brain to support brain health.

Also, during intermittent fasting, the noradrenaline levels in the body increase, leading to feeling full of energy. Intermittent fasting for two consecutive days may increase body metabolism by over 3%. Rather than slow down the body's metabolic state, intermittent fasting can rev it up so that the individual has more energy to move, pending when food is ingested.

Practical Steps to Balance Hormones With the Keto Diet and Intermittent Fasting

Hormonal imbalance has become prevalent due to the fast-paced, modern lifestyles we live. Hormones decline as we age, which also lends credence to the reason for the imbalances in hormonal levels. Hormones have immense effects on individuals' mental, physical, and emotional states. They play a major role in the physical and psychological well-being of individuals, hence the need to constantly balance them.

Balancing hormones is made possible with a combination of intermittent fasting and a keto diet. To achieve hormonal balance, the following should be considered:

Dietary Considerations

Make every meal protein-inclusive: Consumption of protein at every meal is important because dietary proteins provide the body with essential amino acids to maintain bone, skin, and muscle health. Protein also influences the release of hormones that control food intake. Protein also reduces the hunger hormone, ghrelin, while also stimulating the production of PYY and GLP-1, hormones that make you feel full.

Reduce sugary intake: Consumption of sugar, either in beverages of any other form, is unhealthy for the body. Sugar-sweetened foods contribute to insulin resistance and a reduction in insulin sensitivity. It is better to avoid sugar altogether to improve your hormonal imbalance.

Consumption of healthy fats: High-quality natural fats in diets help reduce insulin resistance. Also, dairy fats and mono-saturated fat in nuts increase insulin sensitivity. To optimize the hormonal level of the body, consume healthy fats at every meal.

Avoid overeating or undereating: These two concepts may not be easy to measure, but they contribute to hormonal levels in the body. Consuming too many or too few calories can lead to hormonal imbalance, but this can be mitigated with intermittent fasting.

Physical Considerations

Exercise regularly: Physical activities, like exercise, influence hormonal health. Exercises reduce insulin levels, which leads to a reduction in inflammation, diabetes, cancer, and heart disease. Strength training, such as walking and aerobics, help modify hormonal levels to reduce the risk of diseases and muscle strength loss as you age.

Ensure consistent and quality sleep patterns: Despite what you eat or how much physical activity you partake in, poor sleeping patterns can affect hormonal levels. Even the brain needs quality, uninterrupted sleep to release growth hormones. This is only possible when the body is at rest—during sleep. Sleep for at least seven hours a night to main a balanced hormonal level.

Reduce stress-inducing acts: Emotional health affects hormonal balance in the body. Chronic stress causes spikes or dips in various hormonal levels, such as adrenaline, prolactin, and thyroid and growth hormones. Reduce the body's stress levels by engaging in de-stressing activities, such as visiting a spa or participating in physiotherapy. Relaxation, prayer, meditation, and breathing exercises stimulate the parasympathetic nervous system to reduce cortisol.

To cap it all off, hormonal imbalance is a fact of life and nobody is immune to it. However, the above considerations constitute part of a regimen that can be put into practice very easily whenever hormone balancing is necessary. They are natural solutions that have been tested and confirmed to relieve individuals of symptoms from hormonal imbalance.

CHAPTER 4

WEIGHT LOSS WITH KETO AND INTERMITTENT FASTING

KETO WEIGHT LOSS

Among the impressive benefits of keto dieting is that it helps to ensure weight loss. Many individuals often resort to keto diets when they have unsuccessfully tried other weight loss programs. Various research by health practitioners has confirmed that dietary considerations are crucial to any weight loss program.

A traditional keto diet is aimed at reducing the carbohydrate intake by substituting it with an increased proportion of proteins and fat-based foods. The majority of calories needed by the body are obtained from fat and protein, in opposition to a normal diet with the majority of calories coming from carbohydrates. By reducing the carbohydrate level in meals to less than 10%, the body is primed to enter ketosis, a state whereby the energy source of the body is switched from carbohydrates to fats and the natural ketones produced by the liver.

The mechanism that allows for weight loss during keto dieting is based on the secretion of hormones that reduce hunger pangs (Miao et al., 2007). By reducing the level of ghrelin in the body, the body yearns for fewer calories throughout the day, resulting in weight loss. One study revealed that people with obesity who follow keto diet regimens often report experiencing small food cravings during the process (Cliff et al., 2018). This makes a keto diet an effective strategy for regulating hunger levels.

Another mechanism of the keto diet that causes effective weight loss is the loss of water weight that is a resultant effect of the significant reduction in carbohydrates in meals. When carbohydrates enter the body, they hold significant water. Invariably, a reduction in carbohydrate intake ensures stored carbohydrates are released along with other body fluids—a situation that results in varying weight loss.

To ascertain the relationship between the keto diet and weight loss, expending more calories than you take in results in a calorie deficit. This calorie deficit is obtainable in the keto diet because the calories burned through ketosis increase while the calories gained reduces due to satiety signals. When starting a keto diet, keep track of the carbohydrates that you are consuming. Reducing carbohydrate intake leads to fewer calories stored as glucose and allows the body to enter ketosis quickly.

Eating too many carbohydrates will not allow the body to stay in ketosis since they are stored; hence, the potential for weight loss may diminish. On average, a keto diet of fewer than 50 grams of carbohydrates per day is good enough to stimulate the body to enter ketosis.

The downside of the keto diet for weight loss is sustainability. Following a diet based on a high amount of fat and a low amount of carbohydrates is challenging. The keto diet restricts individuals to certain foods; they may not be used to that, which may make adherence difficult. This may lead to fatigue, poor mood, irritability, constipation, brain fog, and a host of other problems. The challenge of persistently dining out or eating at social gatherings with family and friends affects those who want to embrace the keto diet. Also, the long-term health effects of the keto diet are not yet confirmed; hence, individuals have to consider this factor before starting this diet. However, some negative effects of the long-term keto diet may include an increased risk of kidney stones and an increased level of uric acid, which is a risk factor for gout. Also, nutrient deficiencies may arise from the long-term practice of keto dieting. It is recommended that the keto diet be used cyclically. To alleviate these downside effect, it is highly recommended for individuals to employ a cyclical approach when implementing the keto diet. A cyclical keto diet gives flexibility by allowing individuals the opportunity to increase carbohydrate intake two days a week while following a strict keto diet five days a week.

WEIGHT LOSS WITH INTERMITTENT FASTING

Anyone who knows about intermittent fasting will know that it is sometimes used as a weight-loss intervention. For individuals who intend to shed a few pounds, intermittent fasting is one way to lose weight by restricting calorie intake. The theory behind this is that when you restrict the time allowed for food consumption, you invariably reduce the timing of opportunities to eat.

When engaging in intermittent fasting, food is not eaten for extended periods. The body kicks off a fat-burning system to fuel its energy needs. Patterson et al. (2015) noted that periods of voluntary food and drink abstinence is not a new phenomenon; rather, it is a practice that has been with us since ancient times. Consistent fasting for short periods results in fewer calories available for the body's energy needs. This process will reduce the fats in the body, especially when it is not compensated by eating more during the prescribed eating periods. Any weight loss program is fashioned so that it ensures that calories burned exceed calories consumed, resulting in a calorie deficit. Intermittent fasting also supports this because a large calorie deficit is produced, and these calories are not replenished during the unrestricted period of eating.

Intermittent fasting assists in weight loss because all the food the body needs is eaten in short time periods, leaving no room for snacking between meals. For improved weight loss, the most common regimen involves eating during a 4- to 8-hour window while the remaining 16 to 20 hours are spent restricting any form of food intake. This process kicks off a metabolic process that changes the body's calorie storage capacities, ultimately leading to fat reduction and, subsequently, a significant weight loss.

Equally, it can be said that intermittent fasting is a sure path to initiate the fat burning process that results in the body entering ketosis. This is made possible by the reserve glucose that the body burns for energy during intermittent fasting. Also, insulin levels during intermittent fasting are affected. Intermittent fasting improves insulin sensitivity, preventing weight gain while also decreasing insulin levels—a signal for the body to burn fat. However, eating a little more than necessary and a reduction in physical activity may lead to a recovery of up to 50% of the calorie deficit.

PRACTICAL STEPS TO LOSING WEIGHT WITH KETO AND INTERMITTENT FASTING

The keto diet and intermittent fasting for weight loss are daunting tasks for those who have never engaged in it before. It also may be frustrating as it is quite a lengthy process. Fortunately, some practical steps can be undertaken to get past the difficulties if you want to reach the objective of losing weight:

Get expert medical advice: The first thing to do is to talk to your doctor about your weight loss goal, especially if you have any underlying medical conditions or you are on any medication. Doctors will know if your body system can withstand the rigors.

Know what foods are permissible: Following a keto diet means you will likely not be eating the same foods you are used to. Also, you need to be sure that you can distinguish which foods contains too many carbohydrates that must be avoided at all costs. Kristen Mancinelli, author of *The Ketogenic Diet: A Scientifically Proven Approach to Fast, Healthy Weight Loss,* recommends 30 grams of carbohydrates per day.

Evaluate your fat and protein intake: People often misconstrue a keto diet to mean taking as much protein and fats as one wishes. This is not so. You don't only watch out for your carbohydrate intake; you must also keep your protein and fat intake to a moderate level. Some proteins can be converted to glucose, which takes your body out of ketosis. Avoid "dirty keto" by consuming only good fats and grass-fed and organic plant proteins. Also, avoid unhealthy fats, as intaking too much could increase your risk of heart disease.

Engage in physical activities: It is important to get involved in physical activities, like weight-lifting and cardio exercises such as walking, jogging, or swimming. These activities help burn calories faster while also building your muscle when the body is at rest. If you do not want a muscular body, your weight loss goals are also achievable; just ensure that you take a walk right after the biggest meal of the day.

Choose an intermittent fasting regimen: There are various regimens of intermittent fasting, such as 12:12, 16:8 (lean gains), or 20:4 (warrior diet). You can also try the alternate day fasting, where you fast one day and eat normally the next day, or 5:2 (fast diet), where you fast twice a week while you eat normally the remaining five days. Research all methods to know which one best suits your lifestyle and health goals. You must also consider your work schedule, family life, and workout routines.

Expect side effects: As you embark on a weight loss program through a keto diet or intermittent fasting, be equally ready for one likely side effect—the keto flu. The keto flu is a resulting effect of your body trying to adjust to burning fat for energy. However, not everyone involved in weight loss programs will experience it, as Kristen Mancinelli affirmed in her book. You may also experience some lethargic feelings in your limbs, which may make climbing stairs painful. There is also the likelihood of constipation and diarrhea due to the drastic change in fiber intake. It is important to consume large amounts of pure filtered water enhanced with trace minerals.

CHAPTER 5

ADD MORE FAT-BURNING AND DETOX POWER WITH HIGH-INTENSITY INTERVAL TRAINING (HIIT) EXERCISE

OVERVIEW OF HIIT

HIIT exercises can be described as short bursts of highly intense workouts with periodic rests or low-intensity workouts in between. Examples of such high-intensity activities may include a combination of all or some of the following: jogging, springing, biking, swimming, rope skipping, and knee highs. The essence of this regimen is to engage in any combination of these. Practitioners of HIIT workouts perceive them as quick fixes for people who do not want to spend long hours in the gym and for those who want to lose weight. HIIT exercises have been confirmed to be very effective for burning fat in as little as 48 hours after working out. Recently, a survey by the American College of Sports Medicine confirmed that fitness professionals voted HIIT as the top trending fitness regimen for 2020. These intensity workouts are popping up in various places, promising to help individuals burn fats and detoxify the body in a relatively short time.

HIIT exercises are different from regular endurance workouts because the routine does not limit your body to a particular intensity level; rather, it ignites the body to convert body fats to fuel as you engage in it. Regular workouts will help your body burn fat while you are actively working out. However, HIIT regimens are developed to help your body burn calories, even after you might have finished the workout. This means the fat burning process continues after you engage in HIIT, as you are resting or sleeping. The energy used during short periods of HIIT is more than that of long periods of less intense workouts. This can be likened to the analogy of a car moving steadily from one point to another while another car caught up in short bursts of continuous traffic. It is not rocket science to understand that the latter will burn more fuel than the former, as it does with regular exercise and HIIT training regimens.

The beauty of HIIT is that you can customize the regimen to fit your needs and goals. You don't even have to visit the gym, as it can be undertaken in the comfort of your home or anywhere else. This ensures that no barrier can hinder you from working out—weather, climate, or man-made barriers. One scientifically-tested HIIT regimen is the 4-by-4 from Norway, which involves a slight warm-up followed by four four-minute-long combinations of intense cardiovascular activities; each activity is separated by a three-minute rest period. However, this cannot be rushed into as it can take a toll on individuals with underlying heart conditions and arthritis. Therefore, you may need to consult your physician before starting the HIIT workout.

HIIT has been used in sports, especially by athletes, to increase body metabolism and melt fat faster before competitions. For a cardio workout, HIIT has been the most effective, and it can be performed in a relatively short time of fewer than 40 minutes. The *British Journal of Sports Medicine* affirms that HIIT training, such as sprints and squat thrusts, are more effective for weight loss than continuous moderate workouts, like walking at the speed of 10 miles per hour over a relatively long distance. Also, HIIT ensures that your body releases toxins through sweat. By engaging in HIIT, you are bound to enjoy both benefits simultaneously.

So whether your goal is to reduce body fat or to detox your body, HIIT workouts help you achieve either or both of these. Don't depend solely on diets or intermittent fasting to get the desired effect of fat burning or detoxifying the body. Aside from these benefits, HIIT improves the overall working condition of the heart. As Martin Gibala noted in *The One Minute Workout,* the more aerobically fit a person is, the better the heart pumps blood, leading to a longer time before you get out of breath. Your body stays healthy and nourished, and you develop the strength to endure more physical stress.

PRACTICAL 30-DAY WORKOUT PLAN AT HOME

If you intend to try out a HIIT regime, you should first highlight the particular cardiovascular exercises you most enjoy doing. This will enable you to develop a HIIT schedule that does not put too much strain on you. If you are ready to undertake this workout to burn fat or detoxify the body, try this 30-day HIIT challenge. The workouts here are developed to involve your whole body so that you can get a full-body transformation. It will require a few minutes of your time daily. You will need a mat, an interval timer, and a set of medium-sized dumbbells.

Day 1

Arm and shoulder workout: interval time of 40 seconds of high-intensity activity and 15 seconds of rest. Complete these exercises in three rounds with a 60-second break between rounds.

- Mountain climbers, 20 reps
- Push-ups, 20 reps
- Squat to shoulder press (with dumbbells), 20 reps
- Triceps extensions (with dumbbells), 20 reps

Day 2

Butt workout: interval time of 40 seconds of high-intensity activity and 15 seconds of rest. Complete these exercises in four rounds with a 60-second break between rounds.

- Jump squats, 20 reps
- Donkey kick (left leg), 15 reps
- Donkey kick (right leg), 15 reps
- Walking lunges (with dumbbells), 20 reps

Day 3

Slight body-fat shedder: This fast workout will kick off your fat burning process. Undertake each workout in 40 seconds, resting for 15 seconds in between. Remember to move fast to complete more cycles within the prescribed time. Complete four rounds, with a 30-second rest between each.

- One-legged burpee
- 180-degree jump squat

Day 4

Slight body-stretch: Stretch your muscles to strengthen the joints and give the body flexible motion. Undertake each work out in 30 seconds, with a 10-second rest between each. Complete three rounds, with a 60-second rest between each round.

- Side stretch
- Biceps stretch
- Triceps stretch
- Hamstring stretch

Day 5

Leg workouts: Activate the muscles of the lower part of the body. Undertake the following exercise for 30 seconds and rest for 10 seconds between each exercise. Complete four rounds, with a 60-second rest between each round.

- Squat jacks
- Reverse lunge with a front kick
- Forward-backwards bounds
- Four squat flips

Day 6

Deep body-fat blaster: where the major fat-burning activities start. Each exercise is expected to last for 30 seconds, with 10-second rests between. Complete three rounds; remember to have a 40-second rest between rounds.

- Squat curl
- Dumbbell swing
- Russian Twist
- Lunge with dumbbell press

Day 7

Abs strengthening: workout combo of light weight-lifting and cardiovascular workouts to strengthen the abdomen. Each workout is to be undertaken for 45 seconds, with 25-second rests between. Complete all workouts by going four rounds.

- Mountain climber
- Bicycle crunch
- Weighted side bend (left side)
- Weighted side bend (right side)
- Russian Twist
- Planking

Day 8

Chest workout: targeted at the chest region to give you strong muscular development above the colon. Each workout is expected to last for 45 seconds, with 15-second rests between. Complete three rounds, making sure you rest for 90 seconds between rounds.

- Chest press (with dumbbells)
- Plyometric push-up
- Chest fly (with dumbbells)
- Conventional push-ups
- Straight arm dumbbell pullovers

Day 9

Deep body stretch: targeted to give your body overall flexibility; also an essential component of a strong body structure. Start with a light warm-up. Proceed with each workout for a minimum of 60 seconds and a maximum of 90 seconds. Complete four rounds, with a 60-second rest between.

- Side stretch
- Biceps stretch
- Triceps stretch
- Shoulder stretch
- Quad stretch
- Hamstring stretch

Day 10

Total body tone: includes both cardiovascular and strength workouts. Undertake each workout for 50 seconds, with 10-second rests in between. Complete four rounds, resting for 90 seconds between every round.

- Sumo squat
- Alternating lunge with bicep curl
- Crunch and punch (with dumbbells)
- Planking
- Two-arm dumbbell row (with dumbbell)

Complete this workout every 10 days in three cycles to get a 30-day workout plan. For more information on the procedures for every workout mentioned, there are thousands of videos online to show you how it is done.

CHAPTER 6

As individuals age, there will always be a buildup of fat and toxins in the body. The more these agents compound in the body, the higher the risk of developing health-challenging ailments that impact daily living. The essence of the dietary and physical practices discussed in this book is to keep your physical health at an optimal level while reducing the risk of health challenges. From weight control through a keto diet to body detoxification through intermittent fasting and HIIT, the benefits of the practices recommended in this book are immense.

Now, understand that the journey to good health and aging depends on what you take, when you take it, and the physical activities in which you engage. For many people, especially the working class who engage in sedentary jobs, your physical health becomes even more important as you age.

It is never too late to change your habits and kickstart your journey to an improved lifestyle through a range of physical and dietary practices that will ensure that your body continues to operate at optimal functionality. You may not need to undertake the practices simultaneously;

you may start slowly with dietary and physical activities while you try to inculcate others as you gain more strength and discipline. For example, if you have never fasted before, it is best to start this by simply skipping breakfast or eating a late lunch and skipping dinner.

To get most of the dietary and exercise regimens discussed in this book, adhere to the minimum recommended amount. However, ensure that you talk to your physician before undertaking the recommended activities, especially if you have an underlying health condition or you feel you are at an age where your strength might not carry the rigors of the recommended activities.

The dietary and physical activities discussed are not for everyone. Simply encouraging anyone to take up the practices discussed is not enough; be sure that your body can handle them before undertaking the practices. To start intermittent fasting, you need to figure out which regimen suits you. For example, I use a combination of the 18:6 and the 5:2 regimen, meaning I do a water-only fast two days a week and use the 18:6 feeding schedule five days a week. And during my eating days, I ensure that all the food I eat is consumed between 12 pm and 6 pm. It is important not to eat past 7 pm, or least three hours before bedtime. It is also important to find the best HIIT regimen that suits you from the HIIT workouts listed. For those who want to enter into ketosis, focusing on the quality of food you eat is vital. However, this should also be undertaken after you might have discussed it with your physician, as there is a remote risk of hurting your body by suddenly changing your diet. Your best health is ahead of you. If you heal your body, you will heal your life. To your optimal health, I am rooting for you.

REFERENCES

Cliff J. d C. Harvey, Grant M. Schofield, Micalla Williden, (2018). The Lived experience of Healthy Adults following a Ketogenic Diet: A Qualitative Study. Journal of Holistic Performance. DOI 10.26712/040520181

Deretic, V., Kimura, T., Timmins, G., Moseley, P., Chauhan, S., & Mandell, M. (2015). Immunologic manifestations of autophagy. *The Journal of clinical investigation, 125*(1), 75-84.

Fung, J. (2016). How Fasting Affects Your Physiology and hormones. Available at https://www.dietdoctor.com/fasting-affects-physiology-hormones#:~:text=Over%20a%20five%2Dday%20fasting,complete%20the%20cellular%20renewal%20cycle.

Jackson, W. T., & Swanson, M. S. (2015). *Autophagy, Infection, and Immune Response*. Wiley Blackwell. DOI: **10.1002/9781118677551**

Klancic, T & Reimer, R. (2020). Gut Microbiota and Obesity: Impact of Antibiotics and Probiotics and Potentials for Musculoskeletal Health. Journal of Sport and Health Science, Vol 9, issues 2, Pg 110-118.

Miao Y, Xia Q, Hou Z, Zheng Y, Pan H, Zhu S. Ghrelin protects cortical neurons against focal ischemia/reperfusion in rats. Biochem Biophys Res Commun. (2007) 359:795–800. DOI: 10.1016/j.bbrc.2007.05.192

Thompson, W R (2020). World Survey of Fitness Trends for 2020, ACSM's Health & Fitness Journal: 11/12 2019 - Volume 23 - Issue 6 - p 10-18 DOI: 10.1249/FIT.0000000000000526

Viana, B R, Naves, J P, Coswig, V S, Steele, J, Fisher, J P, & Gentil, P. (2019) Is interval training the magic bullet for fat loss? A systematic review and meta-analysis comparing moderate-intensity continuous training with high-intensity interval training (HIIT). Available at https://bjsm.bmj.com/content/53/10/655

Zhu MJ, et al. AMPK in regulation of apical junctions and barrier function of intestinal epithelium. *Tissue Barriers*. 2018; 6(2): 1-13.

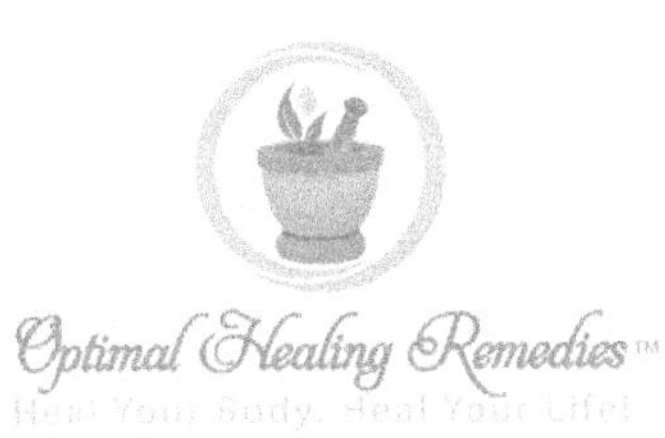

To learn more about how you can heal your body and
your life naturally, visit:

https://www.optimalhealingremedies.com